FitDiary

Volume 1 - Fitness Motivation

By Rita Ferdinando

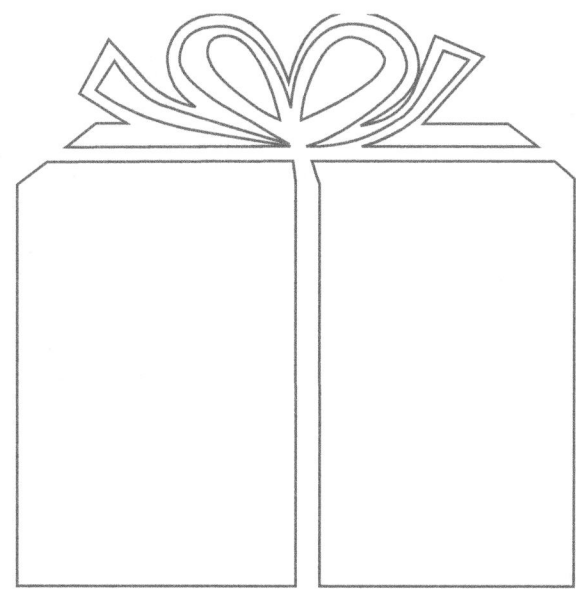

A c k n o w l e d g e m e n t s : *This Book Was Written So That You Will Have The Motivation To Be More Fit And Set Your Goals.*

Fitness Motivation
"Training For Your Vacation"

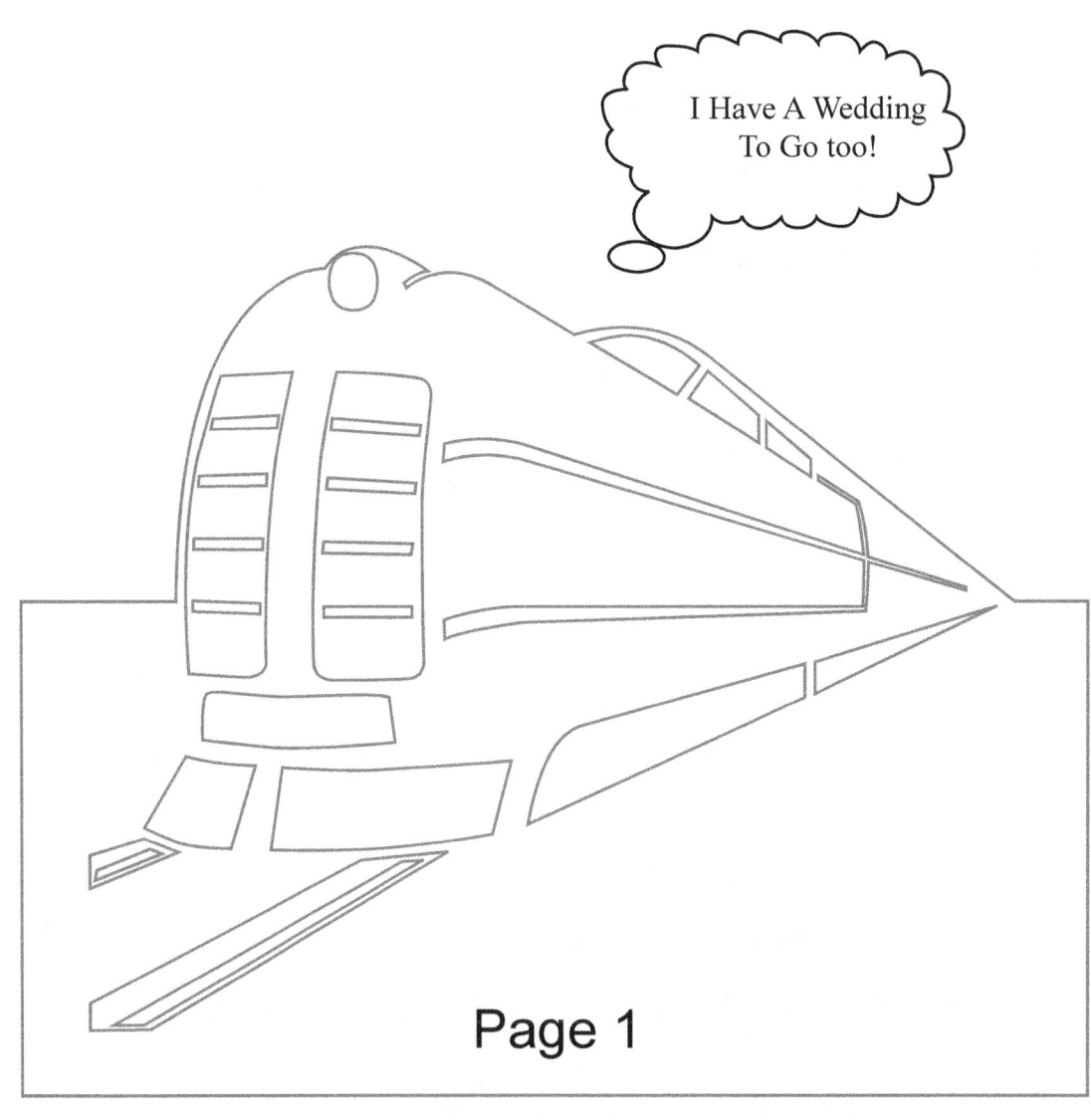

I Have A Wedding
To Go too!

Page 1

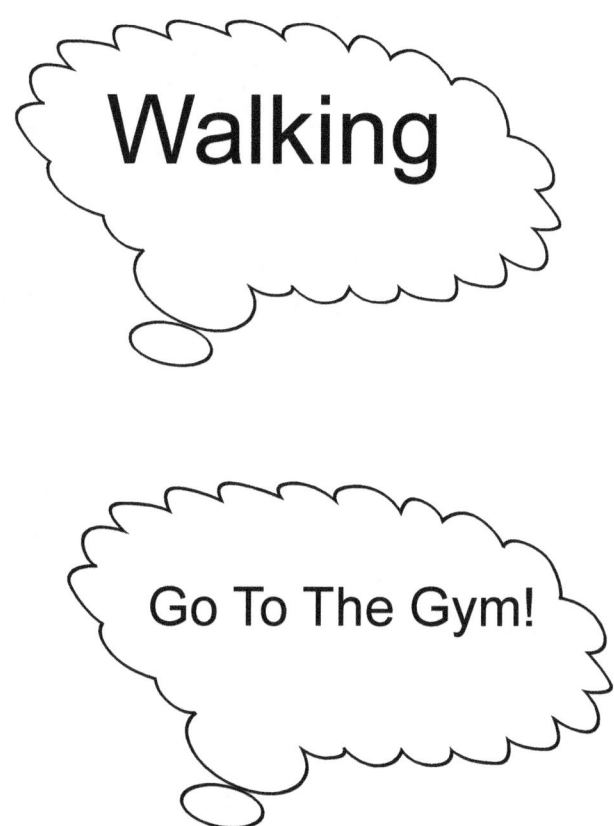

Training Motivation!

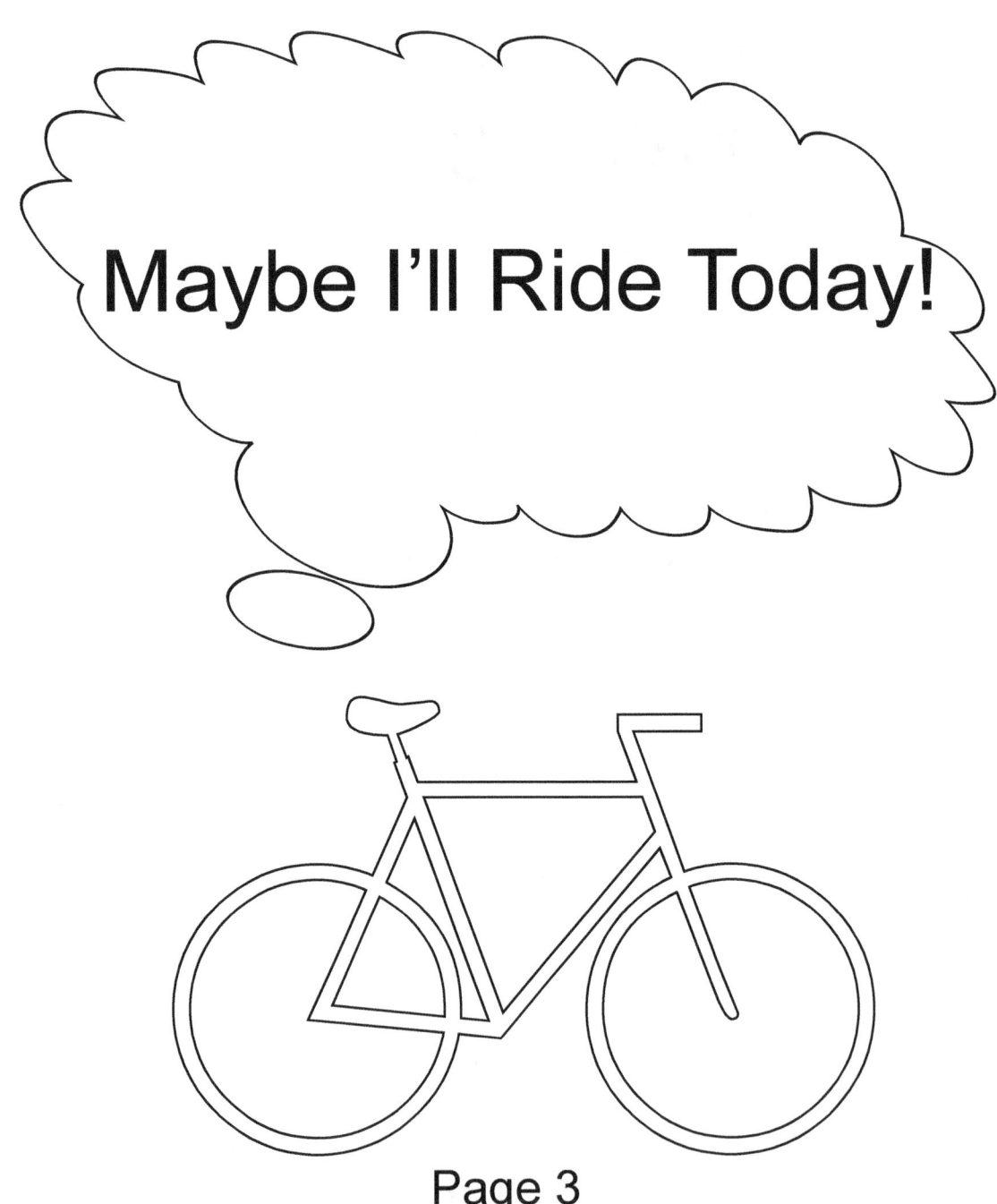

Maybe I'll Ride Today!

Training Days

1: Lets Start Keeping Track
Of The Things Your Doing

2: Weigh Yourself After Work Outs

3: Write Down What You Are Eating

4: How Many Day's You Are Going
To The Gym?

Training
What Did You On Day 1 ?

Your Notes

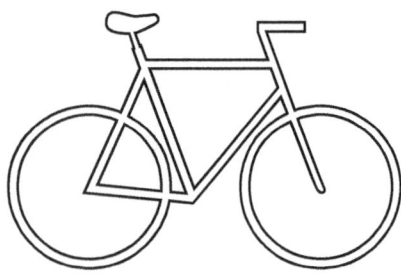

Training
Day 2

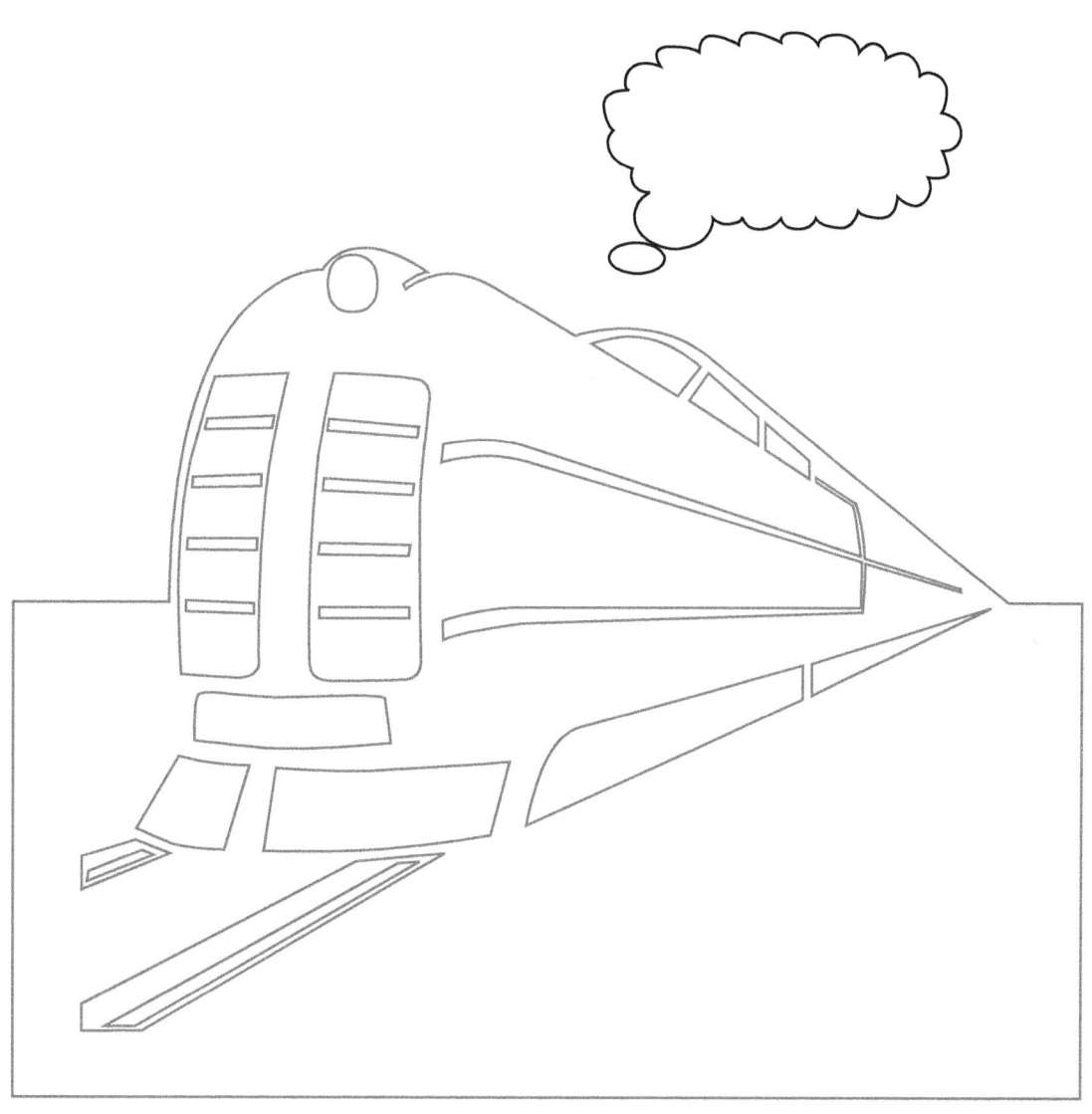

Training
Day 2

What Are You Doing Today?

Training
Day 2

BEFORE WORK
AFTER WORK

Your Notes

$\longleftrightarrow$

What Are My Training Days ?

Monday

Tuesday

Wednesday

Thursday

Friday

Saturday Day

Sunday

Goal is to Train 2 - 3 Day a Week
Consult with your doctor!

Motivation! See Page 25

Training
Days Goals

Your Notes

Training
Days ?

Your Notes

Your Notes

Training
Goals

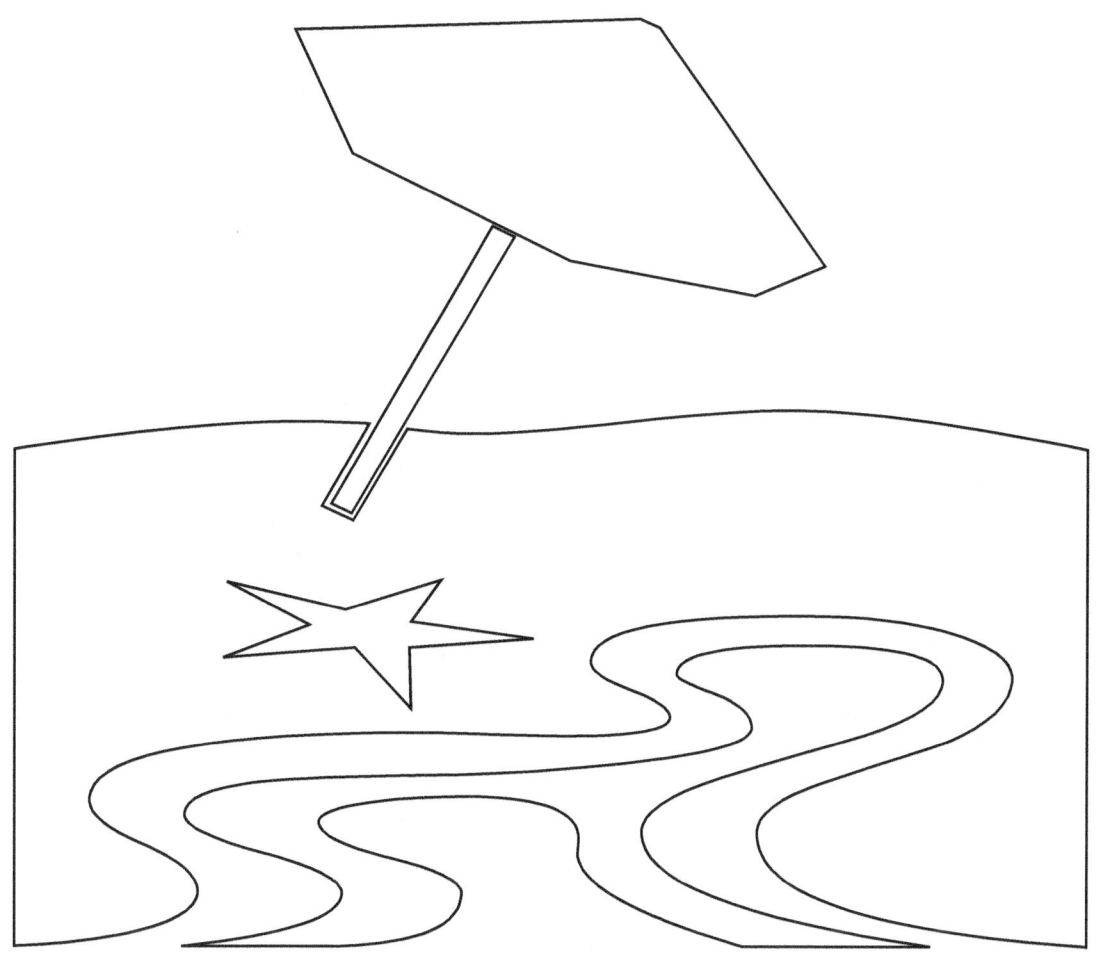

Training
Days

Training Days

Your Notes

Training
Days

Training
Days

Your Notes

Training
Days

Training *Days*

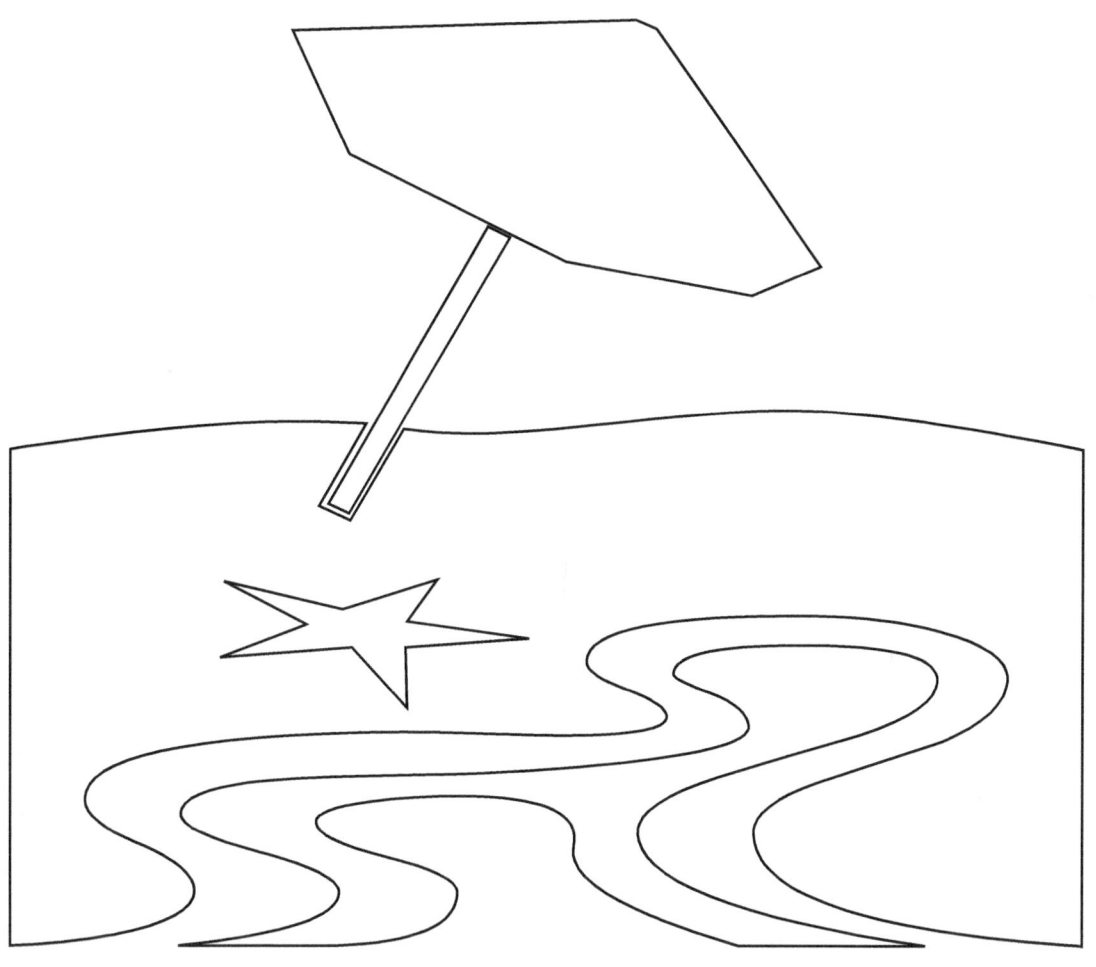

Your Notes

Training
Days

Training
Days

Your Notes

Training
Days

Your Notes

← →

Weigh Lifting
Aerobics
Swimming
Walking
Power Walking
Dog Walking
Golf
Tennis
Bowling
Eating Less
White Bread Or Whole Wheat
What Foods Cutting Out ?

Adding more Fruits or Vegetables?
Found A Work Out Buddy ?
Taking A Class ?

Training

Training
Days

Your Notes

$\longleftrightarrow$

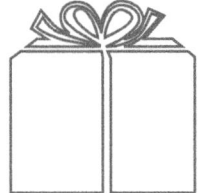 Book Design By Author Rita Ferdinando

TampabayTennisClinics.com